Chapter 1: Understanding Epilepsy

What is Epilepsy?

Epilepsy is a neurological disorder that affects the brain's electrical activity, causing recurrent seizures. These seizures can vary in severity and frequency, and can impact all aspects of a person's life. For family members of individuals with epilepsy, understanding the nature of the condition is crucial in providing support and care.

Coping strategies for siblings of individuals with epilepsy are important to ensure that they feel supported and included in the family dynamic. Siblings may experience feelings of fear, confusion, or even guilt when witnessing their loved one's seizures. It is essential for parents and caregivers to communicate openly with siblings about epilepsy, provide them with accurate information, and encourage them to express their thoughts and feelings.

Epilepsy Uncovered: A Family Guide to Understanding and Coping

Supporting a child with epilepsy in school and social settings can be challenging, but with the right resources and strategies, it is possible to create a safe and inclusive environment. Educating teachers, classmates, and other parents about epilepsy can help reduce stigma and promote understanding. It is important to work closely with school staff to develop a seizure action plan and ensure that the child's needs are met.

The emotional impact of epilepsy on family members cannot be underestimated. Watching a loved one experience seizures can be distressing and overwhelming. It is important for families to communicate openly about their feelings, seek support from each other, and consider therapy or counseling if needed. Building a strong support network within the family can help alleviate some of the emotional strain.

Epilepsy Uncovered: A Family Guide to Understanding and Coping

Effective communication with healthcare providers is essential for managing a family member's epilepsy effectively. It is important to ask questions, seek clarification, and advocate for the best possible care. Keeping detailed records of seizures, medications, and appointments can help healthcare providers make informed decisions. By working collaboratively with medical professionals, families can ensure that their loved one receives the best possible treatment and support.

Causes and Triggers of Epileptic Seizures

Epileptic seizures can be a frightening and overwhelming experience for both the individual experiencing them and their family members. Understanding the causes and triggers of these seizures is essential in managing and coping with epilepsy. There are various factors that can contribute to the occurrence of seizures, including genetics, brain injuries, infections, and certain medical conditions. Identifying these underlying causes can help healthcare providers develop an effective treatment plan to help manage the condition.

Epilepsy Uncovered: A Family Guide to Understanding and Coping

Triggers are specific factors that can increase the likelihood of a seizure occurring in individuals with epilepsy. Common triggers include stress, lack of sleep, flashing lights, alcohol, and certain medications. It is important for family members to be aware of these triggers and work together to create a supportive environment that minimizes their impact. By identifying and avoiding potential triggers, individuals with epilepsy can reduce the frequency and severity of their seizures.

Coping with a family member who has epilepsy can be challenging, especially for siblings who may feel overwhelmed or misunderstood. It is important for siblings to communicate openly with their parents and healthcare providers about their feelings and concerns. Siblings may also benefit from joining support groups or seeking counseling to help them better understand and cope with their sibling's condition.

Epilepsy Uncovered: A Family Guide to Understanding and Coping

Supporting a child with epilepsy in school and social settings is crucial for their overall well-being and development. Educating teachers, classmates, and friends about epilepsy can help create a supportive and inclusive environment for the child. It is important for parents to advocate for their child's needs and work closely with school officials to ensure that appropriate accommodations are in place.

Understanding the emotional impact of epilepsy on family members is essential for building a strong support system. It is common for family members to experience feelings of fear, guilt, and anxiety when a loved one has epilepsy. By openly discussing these emotions and seeking support from healthcare providers and support groups, families can better navigate the challenges of living with epilepsy.

Different Types of Epilepsy

Epilepsy Uncovered: A Family Guide to Understanding and Coping

Epilepsy is a neurological disorder that affects millions of people worldwide. There are different types of epilepsy, each with its own unique characteristics and symptoms. Understanding the different types of epilepsy can help families better cope with the challenges that come with caring for a loved one with this condition.

One common type of epilepsy is focal epilepsy, which is characterized by seizures that originate in a specific area of the brain. These seizures can cause a variety of symptoms, including changes in behavior, emotions, or consciousness. Another type of epilepsy is generalized epilepsy, which involves seizures that affect both sides of the brain simultaneously. These seizures can cause convulsions, loss of consciousness, and other physical symptoms.

Epilepsy Uncovered: A Family Guide to Understanding and Coping

There are also many other less common types of epilepsy, such as absence epilepsy, myoclonic epilepsy, and tonic-clonic epilepsy. Each of these types has its own set of symptoms and challenges, so it is important for families to work closely with healthcare providers to develop a personalized treatment plan for their loved one.

Coping with a family member who has epilepsy can be challenging, especially for siblings. Siblings may feel scared, confused, or even resentful towards their sibling with epilepsy. It is important for parents to provide support and guidance to siblings, helping them understand the condition and how they can help their sibling in times of need.

Supporting a child with epilepsy in school and social settings is also crucial. Educating teachers, classmates, and friends about epilepsy can help create a safe and understanding environment for the child. It is important for parents to communicate openly with school staff and advocate for their child's needs to ensure they receive the support they require.

Epilepsy Uncovered: A Family Guide to Understanding and Coping

In conclusion, understanding the different types of epilepsy and how they impact families is essential for providing the best care and support for loved ones with this condition. By educating oneself, communicating effectively with healthcare providers, and advocating for better awareness and education in the community, families can navigate the challenges of epilepsy with strength and resilience.

Diagnosing Epilepsy in Family Members

Diagnosing epilepsy in a family member can be a challenging and emotional experience. It is important to remember that epilepsy is a medical condition that affects the brain and can manifest in various ways. If you suspect that a family member may have epilepsy, it is crucial to seek medical attention and consult with a healthcare provider who specializes in epilepsy. A thorough evaluation, including a physical exam, neurological tests, and possibly an EEG (electroencephalogram), may be necessary to diagnose epilepsy.

Epilepsy Uncovered: A Family Guide to Understanding and Coping

Coping strategies for siblings of individuals with epilepsy are essential in helping them understand and support their sibling. Siblings may experience a range of emotions, including fear, confusion, and worry, when a family member has epilepsy. It is important for parents to provide information and education about epilepsy to siblings, as well as encourage open communication and support within the family. Siblings may also benefit from talking to a counselor or therapist who specializes in epilepsy to help them navigate their feelings and cope with the challenges they may face.

Supporting a child with epilepsy in school and social settings is crucial for their overall well-being. It is important for parents to work closely with teachers, school administrators, and other caregivers to ensure that the child's needs are met and that they are able to participate fully in school activities. Educating others about epilepsy and providing resources and support can help create a safe and inclusive environment for the child with epilepsy.

Epilepsy Uncovered: A Family Guide to Understanding and Coping

Understanding the emotional impact of epilepsy on family members is essential for providing effective support and care. Family members may experience a range of emotions, including fear, guilt, frustration, and sadness, when a loved one has epilepsy. It is important for families to communicate openly and honestly about their feelings, as well as seek support from healthcare providers, counselors, or support groups. By acknowledging and addressing these emotions, families can better cope with the challenges of living with epilepsy.

Communicating effectively with healthcare providers about a family member's epilepsy is crucial for ensuring that the individual receives the best possible care. It is important for families to be prepared to ask questions, share information about the individual's symptoms and medical history, and advocate for their loved one's needs. By working collaboratively with healthcare providers, families can develop a comprehensive treatment plan that addresses the individual's unique needs and improves their quality of life.

Chapter 2: Coping Strategies for Siblings of Individuals with Epilepsy

Understanding Sibling Feelings and Reactions

When a family member is diagnosed with epilepsy, it can have a significant impact on siblings as well. Siblings may experience a wide range of emotions, including fear, confusion, and even guilt. It is important for parents and caregivers to understand and acknowledge these feelings in order to provide the necessary support and guidance. Siblings may also have questions about epilepsy and how it will affect their relationship with their brother or sister. Encouraging open communication and providing age-appropriate information can help siblings feel more informed and empowered.

Coping strategies for siblings of individuals with epilepsy can vary depending on the age and personality of the sibling. Some siblings may benefit from talking to a therapist or joining a support group to connect with others who are going through similar experiences. Encouraging siblings to maintain their own hobbies and interests can also help them cope with the stress and uncertainty of having a family member with epilepsy. It is important for parents to be patient and understanding, as siblings may need extra support during difficult times.

Supporting a child with epilepsy in school and social settings is crucial for their overall well-being. Siblings can play a key role in advocating for their brother or sister and educating their peers about epilepsy. It is important for parents to work closely with school staff to develop a plan that addresses the child's unique needs and ensures their safety. Siblings may also need support in navigating social situations where epilepsy may be misunderstood or stigmatized. Encouraging open and honest conversations about epilepsy can help siblings feel more confident in explaining their family member's condition to others.

Epilepsy Uncovered: A Family Guide to Understanding and Coping

Understanding the emotional impact of epilepsy on family members is essential for promoting a healthy and supportive environment. Siblings may feel a range of emotions, including sadness, anger, and frustration. It is important for parents to validate these feelings and provide opportunities for siblings to express themselves in a safe and supportive manner. Siblings may also benefit from participating in family therapy or counseling to address any unresolved issues and improve communication within the family.

In conclusion, it is important for families affected by epilepsy to communicate effectively with healthcare providers about their family member's condition. Siblings can play a valuable role in advocating for their brother or sister and ensuring that their needs are met. By working together as a family, siblings can support each other through the challenges of living with epilepsy and help promote understanding and awareness in their community.

Supporting Siblings in Coping with a Family Member's Epilepsy

Epilepsy Uncovered: A Family Guide to Understanding and Coping

When a family member is diagnosed with epilepsy, it can have a significant impact on everyone in the family, including siblings. Siblings may feel worried, confused, or even resentful about their sibling's condition. It is important for parents to provide support and guidance to help siblings cope with their emotions and understand epilepsy better.

One way to support siblings is to educate them about epilepsy. This includes explaining what seizures are, how they can be managed, and what to do in case of an emergency. By providing siblings with accurate information, parents can help alleviate fears and misconceptions about epilepsy.

It is also important to involve siblings in the care of the family member with epilepsy. This can help siblings feel included and valued, as well as give them a sense of responsibility and control in the situation. Siblings can assist with medication reminders, seizure monitoring, and providing emotional support to their sibling with epilepsy.

In addition, parents should encourage open communication within the family. Siblings should feel comfortable expressing their feelings and asking questions about epilepsy. It is important for parents to create a safe and supportive environment where siblings can talk about their concerns and receive reassurance.

Overall, supporting siblings in coping with a family member's epilepsy involves providing education, involving them in caregiving tasks, encouraging open communication, and offering emotional support. By addressing siblings' needs and emotions, parents can help strengthen family relationships and create a more understanding and compassionate environment for everyone affected by epilepsy.

Resources for Siblings of Individuals with Epilepsy

Epilepsy Uncovered: A Family Guide to Understanding and Coping

Having a sibling with epilepsy can be a challenging experience for many individuals. Siblings may often feel overwhelmed, confused, or even neglected as their family focuses on the needs of the individual with epilepsy. It is crucial for siblings to have access to resources and support to help them navigate this unique situation.

One important resource for siblings of individuals with epilepsy is support groups. These groups provide a safe space for siblings to share their feelings, experiences, and challenges with others who can relate. Support groups can offer valuable advice, coping strategies, and emotional support to help siblings better understand and cope with their sibling's epilepsy.

In addition to support groups, educational resources can also be beneficial for siblings of individuals with epilepsy. Learning more about epilepsy, its causes, symptoms, and treatments can help siblings feel more informed and empowered. Understanding the condition can also help siblings feel more confident in supporting their sibling and advocating for their needs.

Another valuable resource for siblings of individuals with epilepsy is counseling or therapy. Siblings may experience a range of emotions, such as fear, guilt, anger, or sadness, related to their sibling's epilepsy. Working with a therapist can help siblings process these emotions, develop healthy coping mechanisms, and improve communication with their family members.

It is important for siblings to know that they are not alone in their experience. By utilizing resources such as support groups, educational materials, and counseling, siblings can feel more supported, informed, and equipped to navigate the challenges of having a sibling with epilepsy. Family members can also play a crucial role in supporting siblings and helping them feel valued, understood, and cared for in the midst of their sibling's epilepsy.

Chapter 3: Supporting a Child with Epilepsy in School and Social Settings

Creating an Epilepsy Management Plan for School

Epilepsy Uncovered: A Family Guide to Understanding and Coping

Creating an epilepsy management plan for school is crucial for ensuring the safety and well-being of a child with epilepsy in an educational setting. This plan should outline specific guidelines and procedures to follow in the event of a seizure, as well as provide information on the child's condition and any necessary accommodations. It is important to work closely with the school administration, teachers, and healthcare providers to develop a comprehensive plan that addresses the unique needs of the child.

When creating an epilepsy management plan for school, it is essential to consider the individual needs of the child with epilepsy. This may include identifying triggers for seizures, implementing a seizure action plan, and providing training for school staff on how to respond to a seizure. It is also important to ensure that the child has access to any necessary medications or medical devices during school hours, and that emergency contact information is readily available.

Epilepsy Uncovered: A Family Guide to Understanding and Coping

In addition to outlining specific procedures for managing seizures, an epilepsy management plan for school should also address the emotional and social needs of the child. It is important to provide support for the child in navigating social situations and addressing any stigma or misconceptions surrounding epilepsy. Siblings of children with epilepsy may also benefit from counseling or support groups to help them cope with the challenges of having a sibling with a chronic condition.

Communication with healthcare providers is key to effectively managing a child's epilepsy in a school setting. It is important to keep all relevant parties informed of any changes in the child's condition, as well as any new medications or treatment options. Healthcare providers can also provide guidance on how to best support the child's academic and social development while managing their epilepsy.

Epilepsy Uncovered: A Family Guide to Understanding and Coping

Overall, creating an epilepsy management plan for school requires collaboration, communication, and a focus on the individual needs of the child with epilepsy. By working together with school staff, healthcare providers, and family members, it is possible to create a safe and supportive environment for a child with epilepsy to thrive academically and socially.

Educating Teachers and Peers about Epilepsy

Educating teachers and peers about epilepsy is crucial in creating a supportive environment for individuals living with the condition. Teachers play a significant role in the lives of children with epilepsy, as they spend a large portion of their day in the school setting. It is important for teachers to be informed about epilepsy, its causes, symptoms, and how to respond in case of a seizure. By educating teachers about epilepsy, we can ensure that they are equipped to provide appropriate support and accommodations for students with the condition.

Similarly, educating peers about epilepsy can help reduce stigma and misconceptions surrounding the condition. Siblings of individuals with epilepsy can play a key role in educating their peers about epilepsy and advocating for their sibling's needs. By fostering understanding and empathy among peers, we can create a more inclusive and supportive social environment for individuals with epilepsy.

Supporting a child with epilepsy in school and social settings can be challenging, but with the right resources and knowledge, families can help their child thrive. It is important for families to communicate openly with teachers and school administrators about their child's needs and to work together to create a supportive and safe environment. By providing information about epilepsy to school staff and peers, families can help create a more inclusive and understanding community for their child.

Epilepsy Uncovered: A Family Guide to Understanding and Coping

Understanding the emotional impact of epilepsy on family members is essential in providing holistic support for individuals living with the condition. Family members may experience feelings of fear, guilt, and frustration when a loved one has epilepsy. It is important for families to communicate openly about their emotions and seek support from healthcare providers and mental health professionals when needed. By addressing the emotional impact of epilepsy within the family, we can create a supportive and understanding environment for all members.

In conclusion, educating teachers and peers about epilepsy, supporting children with epilepsy in school and social settings, understanding the emotional impact of epilepsy on family members, and advocating for better epilepsy awareness in the community are all essential components of providing comprehensive care for individuals living with epilepsy. By working together to educate, support, and advocate for individuals with epilepsy, we can create a more inclusive and understanding society for all.

Encouraging Social Inclusion for Children with Epilepsy

Epilepsy Uncovered: A Family Guide to Understanding and Coping

Encouraging social inclusion for children with epilepsy is crucial in helping them feel accepted and supported in various settings. Family members play a significant role in ensuring that children with epilepsy are included in social activities and not isolated due to their condition. By fostering a sense of belonging and understanding within the family, children with epilepsy can develop a positive self-image and build strong relationships with their peers.

Coping strategies for siblings of individuals with epilepsy are essential in helping them navigate the challenges that come with having a family member who has the condition. Siblings may experience feelings of fear, confusion, or even guilt when their brother or sister has a seizure. It is important for parents and caregivers to provide emotional support and education to help siblings cope with their emotions and understand how to support their sibling with epilepsy.

Epilepsy Uncovered: A Family Guide to Understanding and Coping

Supporting a child with epilepsy in school and social settings involves working closely with teachers, school administrators, and other parents to create a safe and inclusive environment for the child. Educating others about epilepsy and how to respond in case of a seizure can help alleviate fears and misconceptions. By promoting awareness and understanding, children with epilepsy can feel more supported and included in school and social activities.

Understanding the emotional impact of epilepsy on family members is essential in providing holistic care and support. Family members may experience feelings of worry, stress, or even guilt when a loved one has epilepsy. It is important to communicate openly and honestly about these emotions, seek support from healthcare providers or support groups, and practice self-care to manage the emotional toll of caring for someone with epilepsy.

To effectively communicate with healthcare providers about a family member's epilepsy, it is important to be prepared with information about the individual's medical history, seizures, and treatment plan. Asking questions, seeking clarification, and advocating for the best care possible can help ensure that the family member with epilepsy receives appropriate treatment and support. By being proactive and engaged in their care, family members can help improve outcomes and quality of life for their loved one with epilepsy.

Chapter 4: Understanding the Emotional Impact of Epilepsy on Family Members

Coping with Fear and Anxiety

Coping with fear and anxiety when a family member has epilepsy can be a challenging and overwhelming experience. It is important to remember that it is normal to feel scared and anxious when dealing with a condition that can be unpredictable and potentially dangerous. However, there are coping strategies that can help you navigate these emotions and support your loved one effectively.

Epilepsy Uncovered: A Family Guide to Understanding and Coping

One of the first steps in coping with fear and anxiety is to educate yourself about epilepsy. Understanding the condition, its triggers, and how to respond in the event of a seizure can help alleviate some of the fear and uncertainty surrounding the condition. By arming yourself with knowledge, you can feel more empowered and prepared to handle any situation that may arise.

Supporting a child with epilepsy in school and social settings can also be a source of fear and anxiety for families. It is important to communicate openly with school personnel, teachers, and other parents about your child's condition and any specific needs they may have. By advocating for your child and ensuring they have a safe and supportive environment, you can help alleviate some of the fear and anxiety surrounding their epilepsy.

Epilepsy Uncovered: A Family Guide to Understanding and Coping

Communicating effectively with healthcare providers about a family member's epilepsy is essential in managing fear and anxiety. By establishing open lines of communication with your healthcare team, you can ensure that your loved one is receiving the best possible care and support. It is important to ask questions, express concerns, and seek clarification when needed to alleviate any fears or anxieties you may have.

Balancing caregiving responsibilities for a family member with epilepsy can also be a source of fear and anxiety. It is important to remember that it is okay to ask for help and take care of yourself as well. By seeking support from friends, family, or support groups, you can alleviate some of the stress and anxiety associated with caregiving. Remember, you are not alone in this journey, and it is okay to lean on others for support.

Dealing with Guilt and Anger

Epilepsy Uncovered: A Family Guide to Understanding and Coping

Dealing with guilt and anger can be a common experience for family members of individuals with epilepsy. It is important to recognize and address these feelings in order to effectively cope with the challenges that come with supporting a loved one with epilepsy. Guilt may arise from feeling like you could have done more to prevent seizures or from feeling frustrated with the limitations that epilepsy can place on your family member's life. Anger may stem from the unfairness of the situation or from feeling overwhelmed by the constant care and attention that epilepsy requires.

One coping strategy for dealing with guilt and anger is to practice self-compassion. Remind yourself that you are doing the best you can in a difficult situation and that it is okay to have these feelings. Seek support from other family members, friends, or a therapist who can provide a listening ear and help you process your emotions. It is important to remember that you are not alone in your struggles and that it is okay to ask for help when you need it.

Epilepsy Uncovered: A Family Guide to Understanding and Coping

Supporting a child with epilepsy in school and social settings can also contribute to feelings of guilt and anger. It is important to work with your child's school to create a supportive and inclusive environment where they can thrive. Educate teachers, classmates, and other parents about epilepsy to help reduce stigma and promote understanding. Encourage your child to participate in activities that they enjoy and to build positive relationships with their peers.

Understanding the emotional impact of epilepsy on family members is crucial in order to provide effective support. Take the time to communicate openly and honestly with your family about how epilepsy is affecting each of you. Encourage family members to express their feelings and concerns, and work together to find solutions that address everyone's needs. Remember that each family member may have a different perspective on epilepsy and that it is important to listen and validate each person's experience.

Epilepsy Uncovered: A Family Guide to Understanding and Coping

In conclusion, dealing with guilt and anger when a family member has epilepsy can be a complex and challenging process. By practicing self-compassion, seeking support, and educating others about epilepsy, you can better cope with these difficult emotions. Remember that it is okay to ask for help and to prioritize your own well-being as well as that of your family member with epilepsy. By working together as a family, you can navigate the emotional impact of epilepsy and support each other through the ups and downs of the journey.

Seeking Emotional Support for Family Members

When a family member is diagnosed with epilepsy, it can be a challenging and emotional experience for everyone involved. It is important to seek emotional support for yourself and your family members during this time. Coping strategies for siblings of individuals with epilepsy are crucial in helping them understand and navigate their feelings about their sibling's condition. It is important for parents and caregivers to provide a safe space for siblings to express their emotions and concerns.

Epilepsy Uncovered: A Family Guide to Understanding and Coping

Supporting a child with epilepsy in school and social settings can also be a daunting task. It is important to educate teachers, classmates, and friends about epilepsy to create a supportive environment for the child. Encouraging open communication and providing resources for the child to manage their condition can help alleviate stress and anxiety in school and social settings.

Understanding the emotional impact of epilepsy on family members is essential in providing effective support. It is common for family members to experience feelings of fear, guilt, and frustration when a loved one has epilepsy. Seeking counseling or therapy can help family members process their emotions and develop coping strategies to navigate the challenges of living with epilepsy.

Epilepsy Uncovered: A Family Guide to Understanding and Coping

Communicating effectively with healthcare providers about a family member's epilepsy is crucial in ensuring that they receive the best care possible. It is important to ask questions, seek clarification, and advocate for the needs of your loved one. Building a strong relationship with healthcare providers can help alleviate stress and ensure that your family member receives the necessary support and treatment.

Balancing caregiving responsibilities for a family member with epilepsy can be overwhelming at times. It is important to prioritize self-care and seek support from family, friends, or support groups. Financial considerations and resources for families affected by epilepsy can also provide relief and assistance in managing the costs associated with treatment and care. Advocating for better epilepsy awareness and education in the community can help reduce stigma and misconceptions surrounding epilepsy within the family and society as a whole. Remember, you are not alone in this journey, and seeking emotional support is a crucial step in navigating the challenges of living with epilepsy as a family.

Chapter 5: How to Communicate Effectively with Healthcare Providers about a Family Member's Epilepsy

Keeping a Seizure Journal

Keeping a Seizure Journal can be a valuable tool for families dealing with epilepsy. By documenting the frequency, duration, and details of seizures, caregivers can provide healthcare providers with crucial information that may help in determining the most effective treatment plan for their loved one. A seizure journal can also help track patterns and triggers that may be contributing to seizures, allowing for better management and control of the condition.

Epilepsy Uncovered: A Family Guide to Understanding and Coping

It is important for family members to work together to maintain the seizure journal, ensuring that accurate and detailed information is recorded each time a seizure occurs. This collaborative effort can help provide a comprehensive picture of the individual's seizure activity, which can be instrumental in guiding healthcare decisions and treatment strategies. By taking an active role in maintaining the seizure journal, family members can feel empowered and involved in the care of their loved one with epilepsy.

In addition to documenting seizure activity, it can be helpful to also record any changes in medication, side effects, and other relevant information in the seizure journal. This comprehensive approach can provide healthcare providers with a more complete understanding of the individual's epilepsy and overall health, allowing for more personalized and effective care. By keeping detailed and accurate records, families can play a key role in advocating for the best possible treatment for their loved one.

Furthermore, maintaining a seizure journal can also help families track progress and identify trends over time. By reviewing the information recorded in the journal, caregivers can gain insight into how well the current treatment plan is working, and whether any adjustments may be needed. This ongoing monitoring can provide valuable feedback to healthcare providers and empower families to take an active role in managing their loved one's epilepsy.

Overall, keeping a seizure journal can be a powerful tool for families coping with epilepsy. By documenting seizure activity, medication changes, and other relevant information, caregivers can provide healthcare providers with vital information that may help in improving the quality of care for their loved one. This collaborative approach can help empower families to take an active role in managing epilepsy and advocating for the best possible outcomes for their family member.

Asking Questions and Seeking Clarification

Epilepsy Uncovered: A Family Guide to Understanding and Coping

In the journey of understanding and coping with epilepsy as a family, one crucial aspect is asking questions and seeking clarification. It is important to be proactive in seeking information and guidance to better support your loved one with epilepsy. By asking questions, you can gain a deeper understanding of the condition and how it may impact your family member's life.

When seeking clarification about epilepsy, it is essential to communicate openly and honestly with healthcare providers. Don't hesitate to ask about treatment options, potential side effects, and how to best manage seizures. By being informed, you can play a more active role in your family member's care and decision-making process.

For siblings of individuals with epilepsy, it can be challenging to navigate the emotions and uncertainties that come with having a brother or sister with the condition. It is important for siblings to ask questions and seek support from parents, healthcare providers, or support groups to better cope with their feelings and understand how they can help their sibling.

Epilepsy Uncovered: A Family Guide to Understanding and Coping

In school and social settings, it is important to communicate with teachers, school administrators, and friends about your family member's epilepsy. By educating others about the condition and how to respond in case of a seizure, you can create a supportive environment for your loved one. Seeking clarification and asking questions can help dispel myths and misconceptions surrounding epilepsy.

As a family affected by epilepsy, it is crucial to advocate for better awareness and education in your community. By sharing your experiences and knowledge, you can help reduce stigma and improve resources for families facing similar challenges. Remember, by asking questions and seeking clarification, you are taking an active role in supporting your family member and promoting a better understanding of epilepsy.

Advocating for the Best Care for a Family Member with Epilepsy

Epilepsy Uncovered: A Family Guide to Understanding and Coping

Advocating for the best care for a family member with epilepsy is crucial in ensuring their well-being and quality of life. As a family, it is important to educate yourselves about epilepsy and understand the various treatment options available. By being informed, you can actively participate in decision-making processes and advocate for the most effective care for your loved one.

Coping strategies for siblings of individuals with epilepsy are essential in helping them navigate the challenges that come with having a family member with this condition. It is important to create a supportive environment for siblings, where they can express their feelings and concerns openly. Encouraging open communication and providing resources for support can help siblings cope with the emotional impact of epilepsy on their family.

Epilepsy Uncovered: A Family Guide to Understanding and Coping

Supporting a child with epilepsy in school and social settings requires collaboration between parents, teachers, and healthcare providers. It is important to create a comprehensive care plan that addresses the child's needs in various settings. By advocating for accommodations and support services in school, you can ensure that your child receives the necessary assistance to thrive academically and socially.

Understanding the emotional impact of epilepsy on family members is essential in fostering a supportive and empathetic environment. It is common for family members to experience feelings of fear, guilt, and frustration when caring for a loved one with epilepsy. By acknowledging and addressing these emotions, you can strengthen family bonds and work together to provide the best care for your family member.

In advocating for better epilepsy awareness and education in the community, you can help reduce stigma and misconceptions surrounding the condition. By raising awareness about epilepsy and its effects, you can promote understanding and support for individuals and families affected by the condition. By working together as a family and with healthcare providers, you can ensure that your loved one receives the best care and support possible.

Chapter 6: Balancing Caregiving Responsibilities for a Family Member with Epilepsy

Sharing Caregiving Duties among Family Members

Sharing caregiving duties among family members is crucial when a loved one has epilepsy. It is important for family members to work together to provide the best care and support for their family member with epilepsy. This subchapter will discuss strategies for dividing caregiving responsibilities among family members to ensure that the needs of the individual with epilepsy are met.

Epilepsy Uncovered: A Family Guide to Understanding and Coping

When it comes to sharing caregiving duties, communication is key. Family members should openly discuss their strengths, availability, and limitations when it comes to caregiving. By having open and honest conversations, family members can create a caregiving plan that is fair and equitable for everyone involved. This can help prevent burnout and ensure that the individual with epilepsy receives the best care possible.

It is also important for family members to recognize the emotional impact that epilepsy can have on everyone in the family. By acknowledging and addressing these emotions, family members can better support each other and work together to provide a supportive environment for their loved one with epilepsy. This may involve seeking support from a therapist or support group to help navigate the emotional challenges that come with caring for someone with epilepsy.

In addition to emotional support, family members should also consider the financial implications of caring for a loved one with epilepsy. This may involve exploring resources and financial assistance available for families affected by epilepsy. By understanding the financial considerations and resources available, family members can better plan for the future and ensure that their loved one with epilepsy receives the care they need.

Overall, sharing caregiving duties among family members is essential for providing the best care and support for a family member with epilepsy. By communicating openly, addressing emotional challenges, and considering financial implications, family members can work together to create a supportive and nurturing environment for their loved one with epilepsy. This subchapter will provide practical tips and strategies for families to navigate caregiving responsibilities and support their family member with epilepsy effectively.

Taking Care of Yourself while Caring for Someone with Epilepsy

Epilepsy Uncovered: A Family Guide to Understanding and Coping

Taking care of yourself while caring for someone with epilepsy is crucial in maintaining your own well-being and ability to effectively support your loved one. It is important to remember that you cannot pour from an empty cup, so taking time for self-care is essential. This may include setting boundaries, seeking support from friends and family, and prioritizing your own physical and emotional health.

Caring for someone with epilepsy can be emotionally taxing, so it is important to recognize and address your own feelings and needs. It is normal to experience a range of emotions, including fear, frustration, and sadness. Seeking therapy or counseling can be beneficial in processing these emotions and developing coping strategies. Additionally, finding ways to relax and unwind, such as practicing mindfulness or engaging in a hobby, can help reduce stress and improve your overall well-being.

Epilepsy Uncovered: A Family Guide to Understanding and Coping

Supporting a child with epilepsy in school and social settings can be challenging, but it is important to advocate for their needs and educate others about their condition. Communicating with teachers, school administrators, and classmates about epilepsy can help create a supportive and understanding environment for your child. Encouraging open communication and providing resources, such as seizure action plans, can help ensure that your child receives the proper care and support at school.

Understanding the emotional impact of epilepsy on family members is essential in navigating relationships and family dynamics. It is common for family members to experience feelings of guilt, worry, and helplessness. By openly discussing these emotions and offering support to one another, you can strengthen your family bonds and create a more supportive and understanding environment.

Epilepsy Uncovered: A Family Guide to Understanding and Coping

In conclusion, taking care of yourself while caring for someone with epilepsy is essential in maintaining your own well-being and ability to support your loved one. By recognizing and addressing your own emotions, seeking support when needed, and advocating for your family member's needs, you can create a more positive and supportive environment for everyone involved. Remember that you are not alone in this journey, and there are resources and support available to help you navigate the challenges of caring for someone with epilepsy.

Seeking Outside Support and Respite Care

When a family member is diagnosed with epilepsy, it can be overwhelming and stressful for everyone involved. Seeking outside support and respite care can be crucial in helping families navigate the challenges that come with managing epilepsy on a day-to-day basis. It is important for families to recognize that they do not have to face these challenges alone and that there are resources available to help them cope with the emotional and practical aspects of caring for a loved one with epilepsy.

Epilepsy Uncovered: A Family Guide to Understanding and Coping

Respite care can provide much-needed relief for family members who are taking on the primary caregiving responsibilities for a loved one with epilepsy. This type of care allows family members to take a break from their caregiving duties and focus on their own well-being. It can also help prevent burnout and allow family members to recharge and refresh themselves so that they can continue to provide the best care possible for their loved one with epilepsy.

Support groups and counseling can also be valuable resources for families affected by epilepsy. These groups can provide a safe space for family members to share their experiences, receive emotional support, and learn coping strategies from others who are going through similar situations. Counseling can help family members process their emotions and develop healthy ways of coping with the stress and uncertainty that can come with managing epilepsy in the family.

In addition to seeking outside support, it is important for families to communicate effectively with healthcare providers about their family member's epilepsy. This includes being open and honest about any concerns or questions they may have, as well as advocating for the best possible care for their loved one. Healthcare providers can offer valuable information, guidance, and resources to help families manage epilepsy more effectively and improve their quality of life.

Overall, seeking outside support and respite care can be instrumental in helping families affected by epilepsy navigate the challenges that come with caring for a loved one with this condition. By taking advantage of the resources and support available, families can better cope with the emotional and practical aspects of managing epilepsy and ensure the best possible care for their loved one.

Chapter 7: Financial Considerations and Resources for Families Affected by Epilepsy

Understanding Insurance Coverage for Epilepsy Treatment

Epilepsy Uncovered: A Family Guide to Understanding and Coping

Understanding insurance coverage for epilepsy treatment is crucial for families who have a loved one living with this condition. Insurance plays a significant role in ensuring that individuals with epilepsy have access to the necessary medical care and treatments to manage their condition effectively. It is essential for families to understand the specific coverage their insurance plan offers for epilepsy treatments, including medications, doctor visits, diagnostic tests, and hospital stays.

Families should familiarize themselves with their insurance plan's policy on epilepsy treatments, including any limitations, co-pays, and out-of-pocket expenses. It is also important to know which healthcare providers are covered under the plan and if referrals are needed for specialized epilepsy care. Understanding these details can help families navigate the healthcare system more effectively and avoid unexpected costs associated with epilepsy treatment.

Epilepsy Uncovered: A Family Guide to Understanding and Coping

When communicating with healthcare providers about a family member's epilepsy, it is essential to be clear and detailed about the insurance coverage available. This information can help providers make appropriate treatment recommendations that align with the family's financial resources. It is also important to advocate for the best possible care for the individual with epilepsy, including requesting coverage for necessary treatments and services.

Families may also need to consider financial considerations and resources when managing epilepsy treatment costs. This may include seeking out financial assistance programs, researching prescription drug coverage options, and exploring other resources that can help offset the financial burden of epilepsy care. It is important for families to be proactive in seeking out these resources to ensure that their loved one receives the best possible care without incurring excessive financial strain.

Overall, understanding insurance coverage for epilepsy treatment is a critical aspect of managing this condition within a family. By being informed about insurance policies, advocating for the best possible care, and seeking out financial resources, families can ensure that their loved one with epilepsy receives the necessary treatments to lead a healthy and fulfilling life.

Accessing Financial Assistance Programs

Accessing financial assistance programs can be a crucial step in ensuring that families affected by epilepsy have the necessary resources to manage the condition effectively. There are various programs available that can provide financial support for medical expenses, prescription medications, and other related costs. It is important for families to explore these options and determine which programs may be the most beneficial for their specific needs.

Epilepsy Uncovered: A Family Guide to Understanding and Coping

One common financial assistance program for individuals with epilepsy is Medicaid, which is a government-funded program that provides healthcare coverage for low-income individuals and families. Medicaid can help cover the costs of doctor visits, hospital stays, medications, and other medical services related to epilepsy management. Families should check with their state's Medicaid program to see if they qualify and how to apply for coverage.

Another option for financial assistance is the Supplemental Security Income (SSI) program, which provides monthly cash assistance to individuals with disabilities, including epilepsy. SSI benefits can help offset the costs of living expenses for individuals with epilepsy who are unable to work due to their condition. Families can contact the Social Security Administration to inquire about eligibility requirements and the application process for SSI benefits.

In addition to government-funded programs, there are also non-profit organizations and foundations that offer financial assistance to individuals and families affected by epilepsy. These organizations may provide grants, scholarships, or financial aid for medical expenses, equipment, and other needs related to epilepsy management. Families can research and reach out to these organizations to inquire about available resources and support.

Overall, accessing financial assistance programs can help alleviate some of the financial burden that comes with managing epilepsy. By exploring these options and seeking out support from government programs, non-profit organizations, and other resources, families can better cope with the financial challenges associated with epilepsy and focus on supporting their loved one's health and well-being.

Planning for Future Financial Needs

Epilepsy Uncovered: A Family Guide to Understanding and Coping

Planning for future financial needs is an important aspect for families who have a member with epilepsy. As epilepsy can bring about unexpected medical expenses and lifestyle adjustments, it is crucial to be proactive in preparing for these financial challenges. One of the first steps in planning for future financial needs is to assess the current financial situation of the family. This includes taking stock of income, expenses, savings, and any financial resources that may be available.

Once the current financial situation is understood, families can then begin to create a budget that takes into account the additional expenses that may arise due to epilepsy. This may include costs for medication, doctor's visits, therapy, medical equipment, and any other necessary accommodations. It is important to factor in these expenses when planning for the future to ensure that the family is financially prepared for any unforeseen circumstances.

Epilepsy Uncovered: A Family Guide to Understanding and Coping

In addition to creating a budget, families should also consider exploring financial resources that may be available to assist with the costs associated with epilepsy. This may include looking into government assistance programs, grants, scholarships, or financial aid for medical expenses. It is important to research and understand the eligibility criteria and application process for these resources to maximize the financial support available to the family.

Another important aspect of planning for future financial needs is to consider long-term financial planning, such as setting up a savings account or investment plan to ensure financial stability in the future. Families may also want to consider purchasing insurance, such as health insurance or disability insurance, to provide added financial protection in case of unforeseen circumstances. By taking proactive steps to plan for future financial needs, families can help alleviate some of the financial stress that may come with managing epilepsy.

Overall, planning for future financial needs is an essential component of caring for a family member with epilepsy. By assessing the current financial situation, creating a budget, exploring financial resources, and considering long-term financial planning, families can better prepare themselves for the financial challenges that may arise. It is important to approach financial planning with a proactive mindset and seek out support and resources to ensure that the family is financially secure and able to provide the best care for their loved one with epilepsy.

Chapter 8: Advocating for Better Epilepsy Awareness and Education in the Community

Participating in Epilepsy Awareness Campaigns

Participating in epilepsy awareness campaigns can be a powerful way for families to educate themselves and others about the impact of epilepsy on their loved ones. By getting involved in these campaigns, families can help raise awareness, reduce stigma, and advocate for better education and support in their communities.

Epilepsy Uncovered: A Family Guide to Understanding and Coping

One important aspect of participating in epilepsy awareness campaigns is understanding the emotional impact that epilepsy can have on family members. It is common for family members to experience feelings of fear, guilt, and frustration when a loved one has epilepsy. By participating in awareness campaigns, families can connect with others who are going through similar experiences and find support and resources to help them cope with these emotions.

Another key component of participating in epilepsy awareness campaigns is learning how to effectively communicate with healthcare providers about a family member's epilepsy. It is important for families to work closely with healthcare professionals to ensure that their loved one receives the best possible care and support. By participating in awareness campaigns, families can learn how to advocate for their loved ones and communicate their needs and concerns effectively.

Epilepsy Uncovered: A Family Guide to Understanding and Coping

Additionally, participating in epilepsy awareness campaigns can help families navigate relationships and family dynamics when a member has epilepsy. It is common for family members to experience strain in their relationships due to the stress and challenges of caring for a loved one with epilepsy. By getting involved in awareness campaigns, families can learn how to support each other and strengthen their relationships during difficult times.

Overall, participating in epilepsy awareness campaigns can be a valuable way for families to come together, educate themselves and others, and advocate for better support and resources for their loved ones. By getting involved in these campaigns, families can help reduce stigma, improve education and awareness, and create a more supportive and understanding community for individuals with epilepsy.

Educating Others about Epilepsy

Epilepsy Uncovered: A Family Guide to Understanding and Coping

Educating others about epilepsy is a crucial aspect of supporting a family member who has been diagnosed with this neurological disorder. It is important for family members to have a good understanding of epilepsy in order to provide the best care and support possible. By educating themselves and others, families can help reduce stigma and misconceptions surrounding epilepsy within their own circles and in the community at large.

One important aspect of educating others about epilepsy is providing information and resources to siblings of individuals with epilepsy. Siblings may have questions or concerns about their brother or sister's condition, and it is important to address these in an age-appropriate and sensitive manner. By helping siblings understand epilepsy, families can foster a supportive and understanding environment for everyone involved.

Epilepsy Uncovered: A Family Guide to Understanding and Coping

Supporting a child with epilepsy in school and social settings can also be challenging, but education is key. By working with teachers, school administrators, and other parents, families can help create a safe and inclusive environment for their child with epilepsy. It is important to educate others about the specific needs and accommodations that may be necessary for a child with epilepsy to thrive in these settings.

Understanding the emotional impact of epilepsy on family members is another important aspect of education. Epilepsy can be a source of stress, worry, and fear for families, and it is important to address these emotions openly and honestly. By educating themselves about the emotional impact of epilepsy, families can better support each other through difficult times and work together to navigate the challenges that may arise.

Epilepsy Uncovered: A Family Guide to Understanding and Coping

Finally, educating others about epilepsy can also involve advocating for better epilepsy awareness and education in the community. By speaking out about the importance of understanding and supporting individuals with epilepsy, families can help break down barriers and create a more inclusive and supportive society for everyone affected by this disorder. Through education and advocacy, families can help create a world where individuals with epilepsy are understood, accepted, and supported.

Supporting Epilepsy Research and Advocacy Organizations

Supporting epilepsy research and advocacy organizations is crucial in advancing understanding and treatment of this complex neurological disorder. By getting involved with these organizations, families can help contribute to research efforts that may lead to better treatments and ultimately a cure for epilepsy. One way to support these organizations is by participating in fundraising events or volunteering your time to raise awareness about epilepsy in your community.

Epilepsy Uncovered: A Family Guide to Understanding and Coping

Coping with a family member who has epilepsy can be challenging, especially for siblings who may feel overwhelmed or scared by their loved one's seizures. It's important for siblings to seek support from organizations that specialize in providing resources and coping strategies for family members of individuals with epilepsy. By connecting with others who are going through similar experiences, siblings can gain a sense of empowerment and reduce feelings of isolation.

Supporting a child with epilepsy in school and social settings can be a daunting task for parents and caregivers. It's important to communicate openly with teachers and school administrators about your child's condition and any special accommodations they may need to succeed in the classroom. By working together with school staff, parents can ensure that their child receives the support they need to thrive academically and socially.

Epilepsy Uncovered: A Family Guide to Understanding and Coping

Understanding the emotional impact of epilepsy on family members is essential in providing effective care and support for your loved one. It's normal to experience feelings of fear, frustration, and helplessness when a family member has epilepsy. By seeking counseling or joining a support group, families can learn healthy coping mechanisms and gain a better understanding of how to navigate the emotional challenges that come with living with epilepsy.

Advocating for better epilepsy awareness and education in the community is a powerful way to combat stigma and misconceptions surrounding this neurological disorder. By sharing your family's story and raising awareness about epilepsy, you can help educate others about the realities of living with this condition. By working together as a family unit, you can make a difference in the lives of those affected by epilepsy and help create a more inclusive and understanding community.

Chapter 9: Navigating Relationships and Family Dynamics when a Member has Epilepsy

Epilepsy Uncovered: A Family Guide to Understanding and Coping

Addressing Changes in Family Roles and Responsibilities

Addressing changes in family roles and responsibilities when a member is diagnosed with epilepsy can be challenging, but it is essential for maintaining a supportive and cohesive family unit. Family members may find themselves taking on new roles and responsibilities to help care for their loved one with epilepsy. It is important to communicate openly and honestly about these changes to ensure that everyone feels supported and understood.

Coping strategies for siblings of individuals with epilepsy are crucial in helping them navigate the emotional and practical challenges that come with having a brother or sister with epilepsy. Siblings may experience feelings of guilt, confusion, and fear, and it is important for parents and caregivers to provide them with appropriate support and resources. Encouraging open communication and providing opportunities for siblings to express their feelings can help them cope with the changes in their family dynamic.

Epilepsy Uncovered: A Family Guide to Understanding and Coping

Supporting a child with epilepsy in school and social settings requires collaboration between parents, caregivers, teachers, and healthcare providers. It is essential to develop a comprehensive care plan that addresses the child's specific needs and ensures that they have access to the necessary accommodations and support services. Educating teachers and classmates about epilepsy can help create a more inclusive and understanding environment for the child.

Understanding the emotional impact of epilepsy on family members is crucial for promoting empathy and support within the family unit. Family members may experience a range of emotions, including fear, anger, and sadness, as they navigate the challenges of living with epilepsy. Encouraging open communication and seeking professional support can help family members cope with these emotions and strengthen their relationships with one another.

Epilepsy Uncovered: A Family Guide to Understanding and Coping

Effective communication with healthcare providers about a family member's epilepsy is essential for ensuring that they receive the best possible care and support. It is important to ask questions, seek clarification, and advocate for the needs of the individual with epilepsy. Building a strong and collaborative relationship with healthcare providers can help ensure that the family member receives comprehensive and personalized care.

Maintaining Open and Honest Communication within the Family

Maintaining open and honest communication within the family is crucial when dealing with the complexities of epilepsy. This subchapter will explore the importance of communication in navigating the challenges that come with having a family member with epilepsy. By fostering an environment of transparency and trust, families can better support their loved ones and address any issues that may arise.

Epilepsy Uncovered: A Family Guide to Understanding and Coping

For family members of individuals with epilepsy, communication is key in understanding and coping with the condition. It is important to openly discuss feelings, concerns, and questions related to epilepsy to ensure that everyone is on the same page. By having open and honest conversations, family members can create a supportive and understanding environment for their loved one with epilepsy.

Siblings of individuals with epilepsy may also benefit from maintaining open communication within the family. Coping strategies can be shared and feelings of fear or uncertainty can be addressed through open dialogue. Siblings may have questions or concerns about their brother or sister's epilepsy, and it is important for parents to create a safe space for these discussions to take place.

Epilepsy Uncovered: A Family Guide to Understanding and Coping

When supporting a child with epilepsy in school and social settings, communication between family members, educators, and healthcare providers is essential. By openly discussing the child's needs and challenges, families can work together to create a supportive and inclusive environment for the child. This communication can help ensure that the child receives the necessary accommodations and support to thrive in school and social settings.

Understanding the emotional impact of epilepsy on family members is also crucial in maintaining open communication. By acknowledging and addressing the emotional toll that epilepsy can take on the family, members can better support one another and work through any challenges that may arise. Open communication allows for feelings of stress, anxiety, and fear to be shared and addressed in a supportive and understanding manner.

Seeking Family Therapy or Counseling if Needed

Epilepsy Uncovered: A Family Guide to Understanding and Coping

Seeking family therapy or counseling can be a helpful resource for families dealing with the challenges of epilepsy. It is important to recognize that epilepsy not only affects the individual with the condition, but it can also have a significant impact on the entire family unit. Family therapy can provide a safe space for family members to express their thoughts and feelings, and to work through any issues that may arise as a result of living with epilepsy.

For siblings of individuals with epilepsy, coping strategies are essential for managing the emotional and practical challenges that may arise. Siblings may experience feelings of fear, guilt, or confusion about their sibling's condition. Family therapy can help siblings navigate these complex emotions and develop healthy coping mechanisms to support their sibling and themselves.

Epilepsy Uncovered: A Family Guide to Understanding and Coping

Supporting a child with epilepsy in school and social settings can be a daunting task for parents and caregivers. Family therapy can provide guidance on how to communicate effectively with teachers and school administrators, as well as offer strategies for helping children with epilepsy navigate social situations and build strong relationships with their peers.

Understanding the emotional impact of epilepsy on family members is crucial for developing effective coping strategies and maintaining healthy relationships within the family. Family therapy can help family members process their feelings of anxiety, fear, and frustration, and learn how to support each other through the challenges of living with epilepsy.

In conclusion, seeking family therapy or counseling can be a valuable tool for families affected by epilepsy. It can help family members communicate effectively with healthcare providers, navigate caregiving responsibilities, address financial concerns, and advocate for better epilepsy awareness and education in the community. By addressing the emotional impact of epilepsy on family members and working together to overcome challenges, families can build stronger relationships and support each other through the ups and downs of living with epilepsy.

Chapter 10: Addressing Stigma and Misconceptions Surrounding Epilepsy Within the Family

Educating Family Members about Epilepsy

Epilepsy Uncovered: A Family Guide to Understanding and Coping

Understanding and coping with epilepsy can be a challenging journey for families. It is important for family members to educate themselves about epilepsy in order to provide the best support and care for their loved one who is living with the condition. By gaining knowledge about epilepsy, family members can better understand what their loved one is going through and how to help them manage their seizures effectively.

One crucial aspect of educating family members about epilepsy is dispelling myths and misconceptions surrounding the condition. Many people still believe in outdated ideas about epilepsy, such as it being contagious or a sign of mental illness. By providing accurate information about epilepsy, families can help reduce stigma and create a more supportive environment for their loved one.

Epilepsy Uncovered: A Family Guide to Understanding and Coping

Coping strategies for siblings of individuals with epilepsy are also important to consider. Siblings may experience a range of emotions, including fear, confusion, and worry, when their brother or sister has epilepsy. It is essential for parents to involve siblings in discussions about epilepsy and provide them with resources and support to help them cope with their feelings.

Supporting a child with epilepsy in school and social settings is another key aspect of educating family members about epilepsy. It is important for parents to work closely with teachers and school administrators to create a safe and inclusive environment for their child with epilepsy. By educating others about epilepsy, families can help reduce the risk of bullying and discrimination towards their child.

Epilepsy Uncovered: A Family Guide to Understanding and Coping

Understanding the emotional impact of epilepsy on family members is crucial for providing effective support. Families may experience feelings of guilt, helplessness, and anxiety as they navigate the challenges of living with epilepsy. By addressing these emotions openly and seeking support from healthcare providers and community resources, families can better cope with the emotional toll of epilepsy.

Challenging Stigmatizing Beliefs and Attitudes

Challenging stigmatizing beliefs and attitudes surrounding epilepsy is essential for creating a supportive and understanding environment for individuals living with the condition. It is common for family members to encounter misconceptions and negative stereotypes about epilepsy, which can impact their loved one's quality of life. By educating ourselves and others about the realities of epilepsy, we can work towards breaking down these harmful beliefs.

Epilepsy Uncovered: A Family Guide to Understanding and Coping

One way to challenge stigmatizing beliefs is by educating ourselves about epilepsy and the impact it has on individuals and their families. Understanding the neurological basis of epilepsy and the various types of seizures can help dispel myths and misconceptions. By increasing our knowledge and awareness, we can better advocate for our loved ones and promote empathy and understanding within our communities.

It is also important to address stigmatizing attitudes within our own families. Family members may unintentionally perpetuate harmful beliefs about epilepsy due to a lack of knowledge or understanding. By having open and honest conversations about epilepsy, we can challenge these beliefs and create a more supportive and accepting family environment. Encouraging empathy and compassion towards individuals with epilepsy can help reduce stigma and promote a sense of unity and understanding within the family.

Epilepsy Uncovered: A Family Guide to Understanding and Coping

Supporting a child with epilepsy in school and social settings can be challenging due to the stigma and misconceptions that still exist surrounding the condition. It is important to educate teachers, classmates, and other parents about epilepsy to create a safe and inclusive environment for the child. By advocating for better epilepsy awareness and education in the community, we can help reduce stigma and promote a more supportive and understanding school and social environment for individuals with epilepsy.

Overall, challenging stigmatizing beliefs and attitudes surrounding epilepsy requires education, understanding, and empathy. By advocating for better awareness, educating ourselves and others, and promoting empathy and compassion within our families and communities, we can work towards breaking down harmful stereotypes and creating a more supportive and accepting environment for individuals living with epilepsy.

Promoting Understanding and Acceptance within the Family

Epilepsy Uncovered: A Family Guide to Understanding and Coping

Understanding and accepting a family member's epilepsy is crucial for maintaining a supportive and nurturing environment. It is important for family members to educate themselves about the condition, its causes, symptoms, and treatment options. By gaining knowledge about epilepsy, family members can better understand how to provide the necessary care and support for their loved one.

Coping strategies for siblings of individuals with epilepsy are also essential in fostering understanding and acceptance within the family. Siblings may experience feelings of fear, confusion, or even guilt when a brother or sister has epilepsy. It is important for parents to communicate openly with siblings about the condition and provide them with resources and support to help them cope with their emotions.

Epilepsy Uncovered: A Family Guide to Understanding and Coping

Supporting a child with epilepsy in school and social settings is another key aspect of promoting understanding and acceptance within the family. It is important for parents to work closely with teachers, school administrators, and other caregivers to create a supportive and inclusive environment for their child. By educating others about epilepsy and advocating for the necessary accommodations, parents can help their child thrive in both academic and social settings.

Understanding the emotional impact of epilepsy on family members is crucial for promoting understanding and acceptance within the family. Family members may experience feelings of anxiety, stress, or even grief when a loved one has epilepsy. It is important for family members to communicate openly with each other about their feelings and seek support from mental health professionals or support groups if needed.

Epilepsy Uncovered: A Family Guide to Understanding and Coping

In conclusion, promoting understanding and acceptance within the family is essential for creating a supportive and nurturing environment for individuals with epilepsy. By educating themselves about the condition, implementing coping strategies for siblings, supporting children in school and social settings, addressing the emotional impact on family members, and advocating for better awareness and education in the community, families can come together to provide the necessary care and support for their loved ones with epilepsy.

About me

My Name is Stephanie. I have had generalized epilepsy since birth. I had the kind where I just stared at people. Then, at 20, I had a seizure in my sleep. I went to have a heart study overnight. That is when they found out I was having 100-200 seizures (petit-mal). Then when I was 28 I has my first grand mal seizure at work, I was youth pastor and I work at a hospital. My seizures were getting worse when I got pregnant. I was put in the hospital for the last three months of my pregnancy. My family, including my kids, have been my rock, constantly trying to understand and support me in every way possible.